I0816871

STOICISM QUOTES FOR MIND & BODY

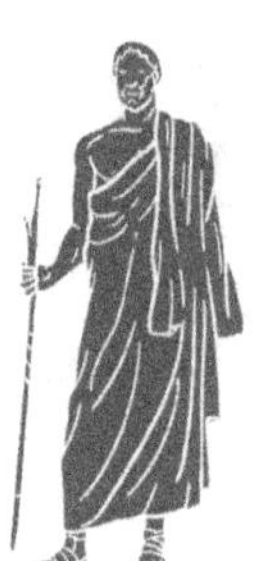

STOICISM QUOTES FOR MIND & BODY

Over 200 Quotations on Health & Well-Being

NICK BENAS, USMC &
KORTNEY YASENKA, LCMHC

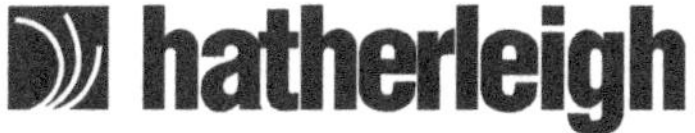

Hatherleigh Press, Ltd.
62545 State Highway 10
Hobart, NY 13788, USA
hatherleighpress.com

hatherleigh

STOICISM QUOTES FOR MIND & BODY

Library of Congress Cataloging-in-Publication Data is available.

ISBN: 978-1-961293-48-9

Cover by Carolyn Casper

Printed in the United States

The authorized representative in the EU for product safety and compliance is Catarina Astrom, Blästorpsvägen 14, 276 35 Borrby, Sweden. info@hatherleighpress.com

10 9 8 7 6 5 4 3 2 1

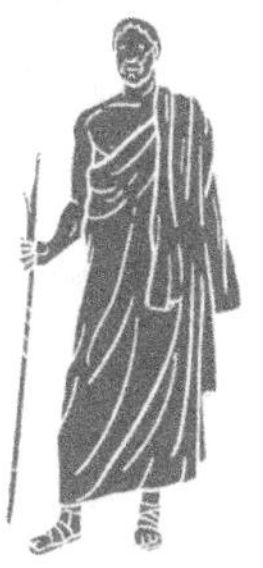

To Hayley Canestrari

Contents

Introduction

CONTAINED IN THIS TRIPTYCH (the third part of a work of art) is a collection of quotations curated from the greatest Stoic philosophers. *Stoicism Quotes for Mind & Body* is the tertiary installment, designed to complement our previous works, *The Stoicism Book of Quotes* and *The Marcus Aurelius Book of Quotes*. We hope that you will be able to refer back to this book often. We explore the following topics: Exercise, Diet & Nutrition, Motivation, Discipline, Longevity, Mental Health, and lastly, Balance. Together, these sections encapsulate the essence of achieving better health and wellness.

The Stoics were philosophers domiciled in Greece from the third century BC, and then later in Rome where they were consumed with gleaning the wisdom of a life well lived. Counsel for those of us struggling with suffering, and the vast, noisy inundation of information. There is a lot of knowledge out there on how to be fit and get six to eight pack abs, yet if one were to glance on a macro level, they would mostly see the rotund. Healthy eating? Replaced with accelerated quick bites, and the processed food poisoning us. Discipline...it's something you don't often see. Motivation? It won't be there if discipline is lacking. If we don't take a hard look at our own lives, our dreams of being pumped up, healthy, and energized will be replaced with great puniness and weakness.

The Stoics suffered great misfortunes and hardships so we could learn. This knowledge is a gift. This is a versatile tool to help us through. Tucked within these pages are utterances from Aristotle to Aurelius. From Porcia Catonis to Publius Rutilius Rufus. From Seneca to Socrates, Cicero to Xenophon, and Epictetus to Zeno. Learn the key to health and wellness from the wise words of these great men.

Zeno of Citium, the founder of Stoicism, is featured on the cover of this book as a tribute to the origins of this timeless philosophy. More than two thousand years ago, Zeno taught that true well-being arises from harmony between mind and body. His vision laid the foundation for understanding that peace is not found in external circumstances, but rather from within us.

I

EXERCISE

Zeno of Citium, who was coined the "founder" of Stoicism spent most of his time walking through his beautiful gardens in Athens. This was his place of respite, for him to connect with nature and recharge. Most of his deep thinking and reflections happened there. The walking and fresh air provided sound exercise and a gymnasium to work his body and mind. The beauty of the gardens stripped away the chaos and congestion of the bustling city streets. The noise pollution was replaced with the beautiful and delicate sounds of birds chirping and the buzzing of bees.

Epictetus, who was born a slave, encouraged his students to exercise to be better prepared for life's challenges. Along with physical exercise, he was an advocate for mental health and self-discipline. Even as a Roman Emperor, Marcus

Aurelius found time to make regular physical exercise part of his daily routine. Musonius Rufus believed in the benefits of hard manual labor. He believed in the benefits of tasks such as digging ditches, much like a Marine or soldier using an entrenching tool to carve out their fighting hole, or a mason carefully laying a marble slab. If one endures the rigors of toiling, the future challenges that are presented should be less laboring. The muscles of the mind and body become exercised and resilient. The results are plentiful, providing better health, more mobility, balance, strength, vanity, and longevity.

STOIC STRATEGIES FOR EXERCISE

Choose Your Activity: Pick a type of exercise you enjoy doing in order to make daily engagement more enjoyable. It doesn't need to be an extremely rigorous activity for you to reap the benefits. Start small and gradually increase the amount of time you spend exercising. For mental exercises, think of Marcus Aurelius, who engaged in daily writing for his own reflective journal, which was not intended for public eyes. Or consider Zeno, who met with friends to engage in civil and philosophical discourse.

Engage With Others: To make committing to an exercise routine easier, include friends or family. This can increase your accountability and make time spent exercising more pleasant.

Change Your Outlook: Being healthy enough to exercise is a privilege. Instead of thinking of it as something you have to do, view it as something you are able to do. See it as an opportunity to challenge yourself.

"No man has the right to be an amateur in the matter of physical training. It is a shame for a man to grow old without seeing the beauty and strength of which his body is capable."

—SOCRATES

"The body is to be treated rigorously, that it may not be disobedient to the mind."

—SENECA

"The greater the difficulty, the more glory in surmounting it. Skillful pilots gain their reputation from storms and tempests."

—EPICTETUS

"It is exercise alone that supports the spirits, and keeps the mind in vigor."

—CICERO

"It has always been a rule that the weak should be subject to the strong; and besides, we consider that we are worthy of our power. Up till the present moment, you too, used to think that we were; but now, after calculating your own interest, you are beginning to talk in terms of right and wrong. Considerations of this kind have never yet turned people aside from the opportunities of aggrandizement offered by superior strength."

—THUCYDIDES

"We ought…to exercise ourselves daily to meet the impressions of our senses… So-and-so's son is dead. Answer, 'That lies outside the sphere of the moral purpose, it is not an evil.' His father has disinherited So-and-so; what do you think of it? 'That lies outside the sphere of the moral purpose, it is not an evil.' Caesar has condemned him. 'That lies outside the sphere of the moral purpose, it is not an evil.' He was grieved at all this. 'That lies within the sphere of the moral purpose, it is an evil.' He has borne up under it manfully. 'That lies within the sphere of the moral purpose, it is a good.' Now, if we acquire this habit, we shall make progress; for we shall never give our assent to anything but that of which we get a convincing sense-impression. His son is dead. What happened? His son is dead. Nothing else? Not a thing. His ship is lost. What happened? His ship is lost. He was carried off to prison. What happened? He was carried off to prison. But the observation: 'He has fared ill,' is an addition that each man makes on his own responsibility."

—EPICTETUS

"It is circumstances (difficulties) which show what men are. Therefore when a difficulty falls upon you, remember that God, like a trainer of wrestlers, has matched you with a rough young man. For what purpose? you may say. Why, that you may become an Olympic conqueror; but it is not accomplished without sweat. In my opinion no man has had a more profitable difficulty than you have had, if you choose to make use of it as an athlete would deal with a young antagonist."

—EPICTETUS

"To summarize: remember that the door is open. Do not be more cowardly than children, but just as they say, when the game no longer pleases them, 'I will play no more,' you too, when things seem that way to you, should merely say, 'I will play no more,' and so depart; but if you stay, stop moaning."

—EPICTETUS

"Take care to be fit, for it is only the body that can allow us to serve the mind, and the mind is the master of the body."

—MARCUS AURELIUS

"Do you not know that life is a soldier's service? One man must keep guard, another go out to reconnoiter, another take the field. It is not possible for all to stay where they are, nor is it better so. But you neglect to fulfil the orders of the general and complain, when some severe order is laid upon you; you do not understand to what a pitiful state you are bringing the army so far as in you lies; you do not see that if all follow your example there will be no one to dig a trench, or raise a palisade, no one to keep night watch or fight in the field, but every one will seem an unserviceable soldier.

"...So too it is in the world; each man's life is a campaign, and a long and varied one. It is for you to play the soldier's part—do everything at the General's bidding, divining his wishes, if it be possible."

—EPICTETUS

"For is not reading a kind of preparation for living, but living itself made up of things other than books? It is as if an athlete, when he enters the stadium, should break down and weep because he is not exercising outside. This is what you were exercising for; this is what the jumping-weights, and the sand and your young partners were all for. So are you now seeking for these, when it is the time for action? That is just as if, in the sphere of assent, when we are presented with impressions, some of which are evidently true and others not, instead of distinguishing between them, we should want to read a treatise On Direct Apprehension."

—EPICTETUS

"Therefore take the decision right now that you must live as a full-grown man, as a man who is making progress; and all that appears to be best must be to you a law that cannot be transgressed. And if you are confronted with a hard task or with something pleasant, or with something held in high repute or no repute, remember that the contest is now, and that the Olympic games are now, and that it is no longer possible to delay the match, and that progress is lost and saved as a result of one defeat and even one moment of giving in."

—EPICTETUS

"Accustom your body to be the servant of your mind, and train it with toil and sweat."

—XENOPHON

"Since it happens that the human being is not soul alone, nor body alone, but a kind of synthesis of the two, the person in training must take care of both, the better part, the soul, more zealously; as is fitting, but also of the other, if he shall not be found lacking in any part that constitutes man."

—MUSONIUS RUFUS

"You must train and toughen your body to serve your mind."

—SENECA

"Everything exists for some end, a horse, a vine. Why do you wonder? Even the sun will say the same. For what purpose then are you, to enjoy the pleasure? See if common sense allows this.

"Pain is either an evil to the body—then let the body say what it thinks of it—or to the soul; but it is in the power of the soul to maintain its own serenity and tranquility, and not to think that pain is an evil. For every judgment and movement and desire and aversion is within, and no evil ascends so high."

—MARCUS AURELIUS

"In the gymnastic exercises suppose that a man has torn you with his nails, and by dashing against your head has inflicted a wound. Well, we neither show any signs of vexation, nor are we offended, nor do we suspect him afterwards as a treacherous fellow; and yet we are on our guard against him; not, however, as an enemy, nor yet with suspicion, but we quietly get out of his way. Something like this let your behavior be in all the other parts of life; let us overlook many things in those who are like antagonists in the gymnasium. For it is in our power, as I said, to get out of the way, and to have no suspicion nor hatred."

—MARCUS AURELIUS

"Everything is born from change."

—MARCUS AURELIUS

"You are well aware that it is not numbers or strength that bring the victories in war. No, it is when one side goes against the enemy with the gods' gift of a stronger morale that their adversaries, as a rule, cannot withstand them. I have noticed this point too, my friends, that in soldiering the people whose one aim is to keep alive usually find a wretched and dishonorable death, while the people who, realizing that death is the common lot of all men, make it their endeavor to die with honor, somehow seem more often to reach old age and to have a happier life when they are alive. These are facts which you too should realize (our situation demands it) and should show that you yourselves are brave men and should call on the rest to do likewise."

—XENOPHON, *THE PERSIAN EXPEDITION*

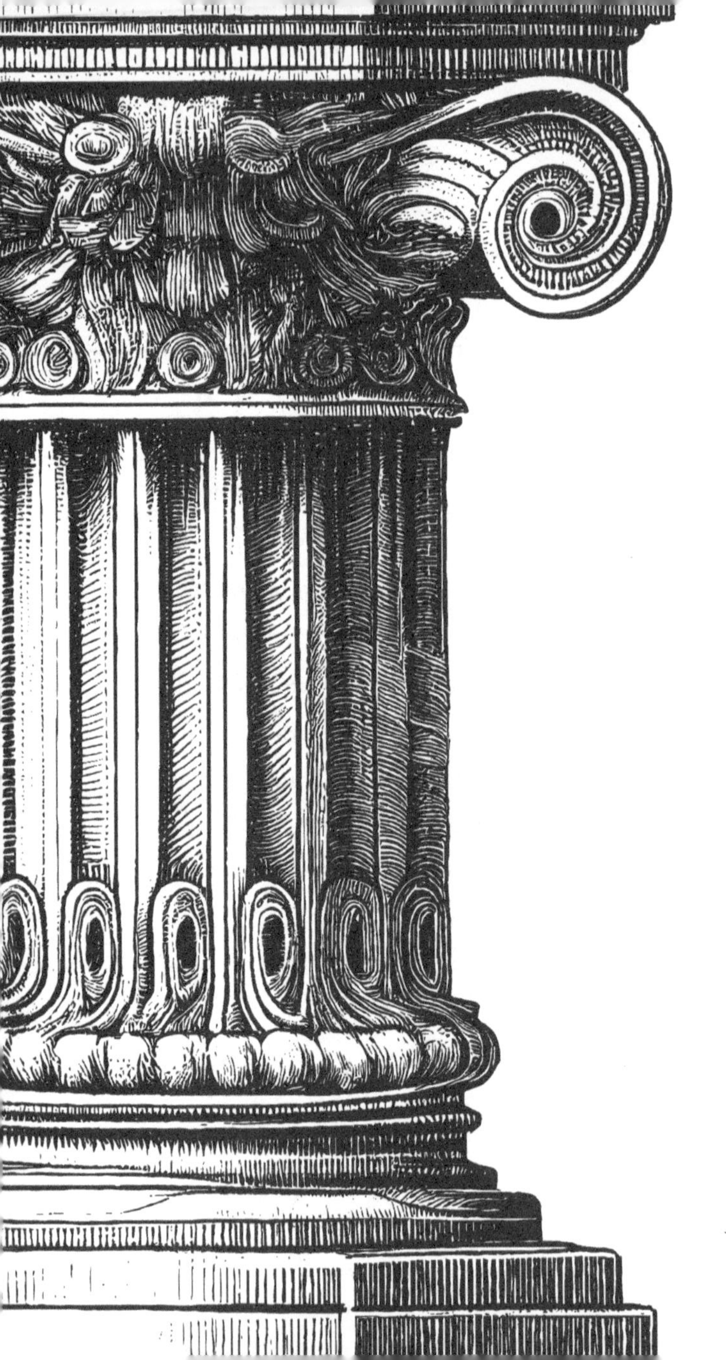

II

DIET & NUTRITION

STOICISM ENCOURAGES A PROPER diet which naturally emphasizes moderation and simplicity. Zeno of Citium was known for advocating a simple diet with minimal luxuries while Musonius Rufus emphasized the importance of sustainable eating by choosing readily available foods. It comes as no surprise that Epictetus, a strong advocate for self-control, viewed eating habits as an act of reason, purpose, and intentionality.

Your diet and nutritional choices should serve a purpose—to sustain the body without overindulging. The key to a Stoic lifestyle is moderation, simplicity, and mindfulness, all of which can be applied to your daily eating habits. Moderation is more about respecting your body and understanding your nutritional needs rather than restricting and counting calories. Being present during meals provides you with a deeper connection and appreciation for the food in front of you.

Seneca was known to "diet" by forgoing the great luxurious Roman cuisine and libations, giving up his favorites of mushrooms and oysters. He also gave up drinking wine. The Stoics believed that those living a virtuous life knew that simple, inexpensive foods were not only healthy for your body but also good for the mind. This approach to diet and nutrition offers useful perspectives on how to approach eating in a mindful, balanced, and disciplined way. Following the eating philosophy of the Stoics will allow you to gain more balance in your lifestyle choices while enhancing your overall well-being.

STOIC STRATEGIES FOR DIET & NUTRITION

Sensory Eating: Appreciate your food and take the time to notice the texture, taste, smell, and beauty of your food. Slow down and view eating as something to be enjoyed, not rushed.

Choose Local Ingredients: Plan your meals based on food that is in season and easy to find close to home. This promotes fresher food and reduces any negative environmental impact.

View Food as Fuel: Be purposeful in your meal planning and intentionally choose foods that are nutrient-dense and good for your body and brain. Eating a well-balanced diet has profound effects on your well-being and ability to regulate your mood and emotions.

"The body is a community made up of its innumerable cells or inhabitants."

—MARCUS AURELIUS

"Let food be thy medicine and medicine be thy food."

—HIPPOCRATES

"He who eats with most pleasure is he who least requires sauce."

—SENECA

"We should eat to live, not live to eat."

—SOCRATES

"Nothing great is created suddenly, any more than a bunch of grapes or a fig. If you tell me that you desire a fig, I answer you that there must be time. Let it first blossom, then bear fruit, then ripen."

—EPICTETUS

"Virtue is the health of the soul."

—ARISTOTLE

"Enjoy present pleasures in such a way as not to injure future ones."

—SENECA

"The best seasoning for food is hunger."

—SOCRATES

"That which has grown from the earth to the earth, but that which has sprung from heavenly seed, back to the heavenly realm returns. This is either dissolution of the mutual involution of the atoms, or a similar dispersion of the unsentient elements."

—MARCUS AURELIUS

"I shall show you a love potion without a drug, without a herb; without the incantation of any sorceress: if you want to be loved, love."

—SENECA

"With food and drinks and cunning magic arts turning the channel's course to 'scape from death. The breeze which heaven has sent. We must endure, and toil without complaining."

—MARCUS AURELIUS

"If you have a garden and a library, you have everything you need."

—CICERO

"Healing is a matter of time, but it is sometimes also a matter of opportunity."

—HIPPOCRATES

"You become what you give your attention to."

—EPICTETUS

"Bitter are the roots of study, but how sweet their fruit."

—CATO

"One man is worth a thousand if he is extraordinary."

—HERACLITUS

"There is truth in wine and children"

—PLATO, *SYMPOSIUM/PHAEDRUS*

"The goal of life is living in agreement with nature."

—ZENO OF CITIUM

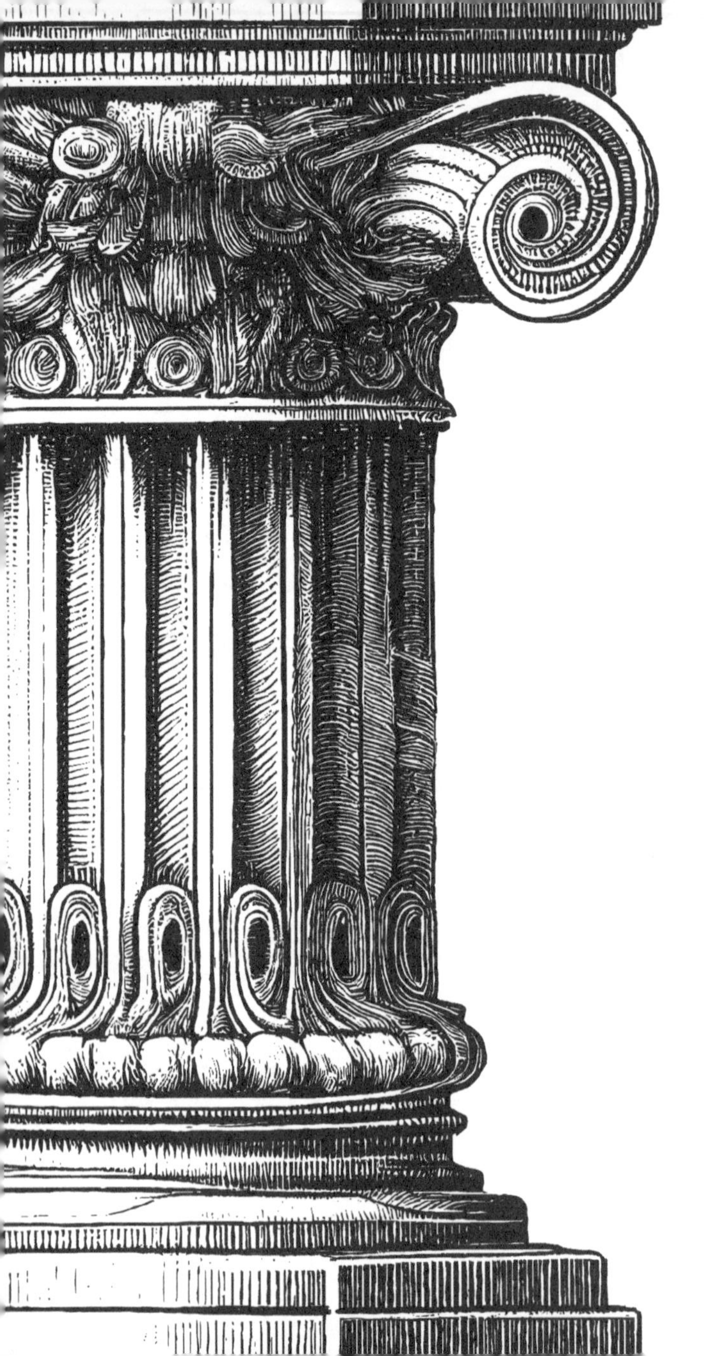

III

MOTIVATION

Motivation is defined as the reason or reasons for acting or behaving in a particular way as well as the general desire or willingness to do something. But what causes one person to be more motivated than another? What causes lack of motivation and what can be done to increase your level of motivation?

While traditional motivation often focuses on external rewards, desires, or emotional highs, Stoicism is about inner drive and mental strength. The Stoic mindset is a valuable tool to help motivate you through all of life's experiences. By encouraging a lifestyle rich in resilience, clarity, and purpose, adhering to the philosophical teachings of Stoicism leads to a higher level of motivation.

Stoics believe the highest good is living a life rooted in wisdom, courage, justice, and temperance. Motivation is derived from the pursuit of these virtues rather than external rewards or recognition. This shift in focus makes motivation longer lasting, as its focus is on internal values rather than fleeting outcomes. Incorporate Stoicism into your daily routine to assist you in building long-term habits that help establish and maintain motivation.

STOIC STRATEGIES FOR MOTIVATION

Establish a Routine: Consistency is key and will help you maintain healthy habits if you commit to regularly taking part in certain behaviors that better your overall well-being.

Start Early: Begin each day with a purpose while practicing gratitude and appreciation. Morning hours are the best for self-reflection and journaling.

Set Goals: Knowing what you want to achieve and having concrete steps on how to accomplish your goals will help structure your day and help maintain motivation. It's best to identify clear and specific goals that are manageable and realistic.

"The impediment to action advances action. What stands in the way becomes the way."

—MARCUS AURELIUS

"Remember that you are an actor in a play, which is as the author [i.e., God] wants it to be: short, if he wants it to be short; long, if he wants it to be long. If he wants you to act a poor man, a cripple, a public official, or a private person, see that you act it with skill. For it is your job to act well the part that is assigned to you; but to choose it is another's."

—EPICTETUS

"If it is not right, do not do it; if it is not true, do not say it."

—MARCUS AURELIUS

"First say to yourself what you would be; and then do what you have to do."

—EPICTETUS

"Waste no more time arguing what a good man should be. Be one."

—MARCUS AURELIUS

"The willing are led by fate, the reluctant are dragged."

—UNNAMED GREEK, STOIC PHILOSOPHER OF ASSOS

"This is the position and character of a layman: He never looks for either help or harm from himself, but only from externals. This is the position and character of the philosopher: He looks for all his help or harm from himself."

—EPICTETUS

"He who fears death will never do anything worthy of a man who is alive."

—SENECA

"There is a story that while Socrates was in prison, awaiting his death, he heard a man sing skillfully a song by the lyric poet Stesichoros, and begged him to teach it to him before it was too late, and when the musician asked why, Socrates replied, 'I want to die knowing one thing more.'"

—AMMIANUS MARCELLINUS

"Signs of one who is making progress are: He censures no one, praises no one, blames no one, finds fault with no one, says nothing about himself as though he were somebody or knew something. When he is hampered or prevented, he blames himself. And if anyone compliments him, he smiles to himself at the person complimenting; while if anyone censures him, he makes no defense. He goes about like an invalid, being careful not to disturb, before it has grown firm, any part which is getting well. He has put away from himself every desire, and has transferred his aversion to those things only, of what is under our control [eph' hêmin], which are contrary to nature. He exercises no pronounced choice in regard to anything. If he gives the appearance of being foolish or ignorant he does not care. In a word, he keeps guard against himself as though he were his own enemy lying in wait."

—EPICTETUS

"It's not possible to live well today...unless you treat it as your last day."

—MUSONIUS RUFUS

"People walk in wickedness all their lives or, at any rate, for the greater part of it. If they ever attain to virtue, it is late and at the very sunset of their days"

—CLEANTHES

"Crimes often return to their teacher."

—SENECA

"What progress, you ask, have I made? I have begun to be a friend to myself."

—HECATO OF RHODES

"There is in fact no way of correcting wrongdoing in those who think that the height of virtue consists in the execution of their will."

—AMMIANUS MARCELLINUS

IV

DISCIPLINE

THE GREEK PHILOSOPHER EPICTETUS was born into slavery in Hierapolis, now known as Pamukkale in modern-day Turkey. His cruel master granted him the opportunity to study Stoicism, under the renowned teacher Gaia Musonius Rufus. This was a remarkable gift, though it came alongside the trauma of being a slave and the injury to his leg that Epictetus endured. It was reported that his master snapped his leg. His education and residual leg limp stayed with him throughout his life.

Epictetus had the self-reliance and obedience to learn under an incredible teacher of philosophy. His teacher Rufus was considered the Roman Socrates, with commitment being the pillar in his teachings. This was later made clear in Epictetus' maturation and prolific work as a teacher of stoicism. When Epictetus later became a free man, it was evident that his discipline carried over into his new life just like the discipline that was exercised in his subjugation as a slave. He gave many talks in Rome, until 93 AD when philosophy was banned in the country by Roman Emperor Domitian. Most of the philosophers fled, including Epictetus who found his way to Nicopolis Greece. Many from Rome and all over flocked to attend his new school of philosophy. He was the epitome of a teacher, embodying discipline in every way. He understood the instant and willful obedience in living and surviving. He also had the self-reliance to continue to learn despite his circumstances. The students knew that. He said, "No man is free who is not master of himself."

STOIC STRATEGIES FOR DISCIPLINE

Understand Your Power: Clearly define what is within your control and focus only on those things while letting go of what is not. Direct your time and energy to aspects of your life that you are able to directly influence and impact.

Emotional Regulation: Attempt to always use rational thinking and reason before reacting. Don't allow your emotions to get the best of you. Practice regulating your emotional responses to help decrease impulsivity.

Focus on Virtue: Seek to embody wisdom, justice, temperance, and courage with every action. Refer to these Stoic virtues to guide your decision making, interactions with others, and life choices.

"He who lives in harmony with himself lives in harmony with the universe."

—MARCUS AURELIUS

"First say to yourself what you would be; and then do what you have to do."

—EPICTETUS

"The soul becomes dyed with the color of its thoughts."

—MARCUS AURELIUS

"Man conquers the world by conquering himself."

—ZENO OF CITIUM

"The more we value things outside our control, the less control we have."

—EPICTETUS

"Habit is stronger than nature."

—QUINTUS CURTIUS RUFUS

"There are three areas of study, in which a person who is going to be good and noble must be trained. That concerning desires and aversions, so that he may never fail to get what he desires nor fall into what he would avoid. That concerning the impulse to act and not to act, and, in general, appropriate behaviour; so that he may act in an orderly manner and after due consideration, and not carelessly. The third is concerned with freedom from deception and hasty judgement, and, in general, whatever is connected with assent."

—EPICTETUS

"Well-being is attained little by little, and nevertheless is no little thing itself."

—ZENO OF CITIUM

"Of these [three areas of study], the principle, and most urgent, is that which has to do with the passions; for these are produced in no other way than by the disappointment of our desires, and the incurring of our aversions. It is this that introduces disturbances, tumults, misfortunes, and calamities; and causes sorrow, lamentation and envy; and renders us envious and jealous, and thus incapable of listening to reason."

—EPICTETUS

"Wisdom is the knowledge of what things must be done, what must not be done and what is neither, or appropriate acts."

—ARIUS DIDYMUS

"The [second area of study] has to do with appropriate action. For I should not be unfeeling like a statue, but should preserve my natural and acquired relations as a man who honours the gods, as a son, as a brother, as a father, as a citizen."

—EPICTETUS

"For industriousness is a disposition able to accomplish unhesitatingly what is benefiting through toil, and none of the worthless are unhesitating with regard to toil."

—ARIUS DIDYMUS

"When you are about to undertake some action, remind yourself what sort of action it is. If you are going out for a bath, put before your mind what commonly happens at the baths: some people splashing you, some people jostling, others being abusive, and others stealing. So you will undertake this action more securely if you say to yourself, 'I want to have a bath and also to keep my choice [prohairesis] in harmony with nature.' And do likewise in everything you undertake. So, if anything gets in your way when you are having your bath, you will be ready to say, 'I wanted not only to have a bath but also to keep my choice [prohairesis] in harmony with nature; and I shall not keep it so if I get angry at what happens."

—EPICTETUS

"Appropriate acts are in general measured by the relations they are concerned with. 'He is your father.' This means that you are called upon to take care of him, give way to him in all things, bear with him if he reviles or strikes you.

'But he is a bad father.'

Well, have you any natural claim to a good father? No, only to a father.

'My brother wrongs me.' Be careful then to maintain the relation you hold to him, and do not consider what he does, but what you must do if your purpose is to keep in accord with nature."

—EPICTETUS

"Better to do a little well than a great deal badly."

—SOCRATES

"For a man to conquer himself is the first and noblest of all victories."

—PLATO

"It is greed to do all the talking but to not want to listen at all."

—DEMOCRITUS

"As fire tests gold, so misfortunate tests brave men."

—SENECA

"He who laughs at himself never runs out of things to laugh at."

—EPICTETUS

"A fool is known by his speech; and a wise man by silence."

—PYTHAGORAS

"Look back over the past, with its changing empires that rose and fell, and you can foresee the future too."

—MARCUS AURELIUS

"Be tolerant with others and strict with yourself."

—MARCUS AURELIUS

"Difficulties strengthen the mind, as labor does the body."

—SENECA

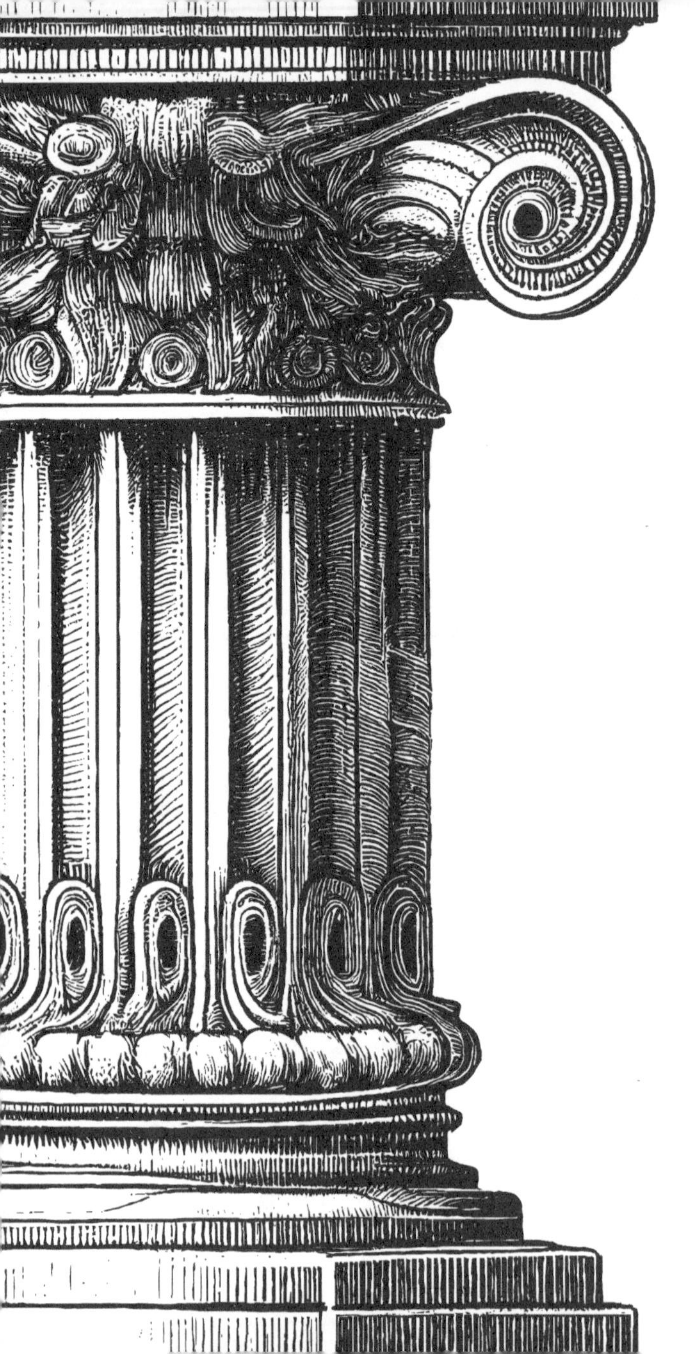

V

LONGEVITY

THE WORDS OF THE ancient Stoic philosophers show their keen awareness that death is a part of life and should be treated with the same significance and importance of living. Since it's a natural part of life, it should be accepted and respected. No one lives forever and time spent on this earth should be of value and purpose. The Stoic mindset ignites a passion for living by reminding you time is precious, and you should act accordingly.

Stoicism helps you focus on the quality of your life and helps build habits that contribute to a fulfilling existence, all of which can indirectly promote a longer, healthier life. It offers a mindset that leads to better overall well-being. By cultivating mental resilience, practicing moderation, accepting death, and living with purpose, you set the foundation for not only a longer life but a more meaningful one. The Stoic mindset helps remove unnecessary stress, encourages virtuous actions, and creates a sense of calm. All of which are conducive to both mental and physical wellness over time.

Epictetus, Marcus Aurelius, and Seneca all make it a point to address the seriousness of appreciating life and being grateful for all aspects of it, even life's challenges and setbacks. To fully accept life, you must also accept death. By following the teachings of Stoicism, you can learn to live more intentionally, appreciate the present, and focus on what matters most to you.

STOIC STRATEGIES FOR LONGEVITY

Prioritize: Examine your life and figure out what is most important to you and your overall well-being. Make it a point to prioritize those aspects of life. Remember you are in control of how much time and energy you give to things.

Be Present: Be mindful and fully immerse yourself in the present. Try to avoid distractions as much as possible and appreciate not only the big things in life but also the little moments that happen daily.

Practice Gratitude: Be grateful for each day and what this world has to offer. Seek to find the good in situations and express gratitude for all aspects of your life.

"No man can have a peaceful life who thinks too much about lengthening it."

—SENECA

"It is not the length of life, but the depth of life."

—SENECA

"Your days are numbered. Use them to throw open the windows of your soul to the sun. If you do not, the sun will soon set, and you with it."

—MARCUS AURELIUS

"What then is that which is able to conduct a man? One thing and only one, philosophy. But this consists in keeping the daemon within a man free from violence and unharmed, superior to pains and pleasures, doing nothing without purpose, nor yet falsely and with hypocrisy, not feeling the need of another man's doing or not doing anything; and besides, accepting all that happens, and all that is allotted, as coming from thence, wherever it is, from whence he himself came; and, finally, waiting for death with a cheerful mind, as being nothing else than a dissolution of the elements of which every living being is compounded. But if there is no harm to the elements themselves in each continually changing into another, why should a man have any apprehension about the change and dissolution of all the elements? For it is according to nature, and nothing is evil which is according to nature."

—MARCUS AURELIUS

"Begin at once to live, and count each separate day as a separate life."

—SENECA

"The whole future lies in uncertainty: live immediately."

—SENECA

"Life is not a journey to be rushed, but a journey to be savored."

—SENECA

"Consider yourself to be dead, and to have completed your life up to the present time; and live according to nature the remainder which is allowed you."

—MARCUS AURELIUS

"Not how long, but how well you have lived is the main thing."

—SENECA

"Wait for the wisest of all counselors: time."

—PERICLES

"Life is long if you know how to use it."

—SENECA

"With regard to whatever objects give you delight, are useful, or are deeply loved, remember to tell yourself of what general nature they are, beginning from the most insignificant things. If, for example, you are fond of a specific ceramic cup, remind yourself that it is only ceramic cups in general of which you are fond. Then, if it breaks, you will not be disturbed. If you kiss your child, or your wife, say that you only kiss things which are human, and thus you will not be disturbed if either of them dies."

—MARCUS AURELIUS

"Life is short, but it is wide."

—SENECA

"Life is a play that does not allow testing. So, sing, cry, dance, laugh and live intensely, before the curtain closes and the piece ends with no applause."

—SENECA

"You should reach the limits of virtue before you cross the border of death."

—SPARTAN PROVERB

"Life is not about waiting for the storm to pass, but about learning to dance in the rain."

—SENECA

"Mortal as I am, I know that I am born for a day. But when I follow at my pleasure the serried multitude of the stars in their circular course, my feet no longer touch the earth."

—PTOLEMY

"Life is long if you know how to use it."

—SENECA

"Nature bore us related to one another... She instilled in us a mutual love and made us compatible...Let us hold everything in common; we stem from a common source. Our fellowship is very similar to an arch of stones, which would fall apart, if they did not reciprocally support each other."

—SENECA

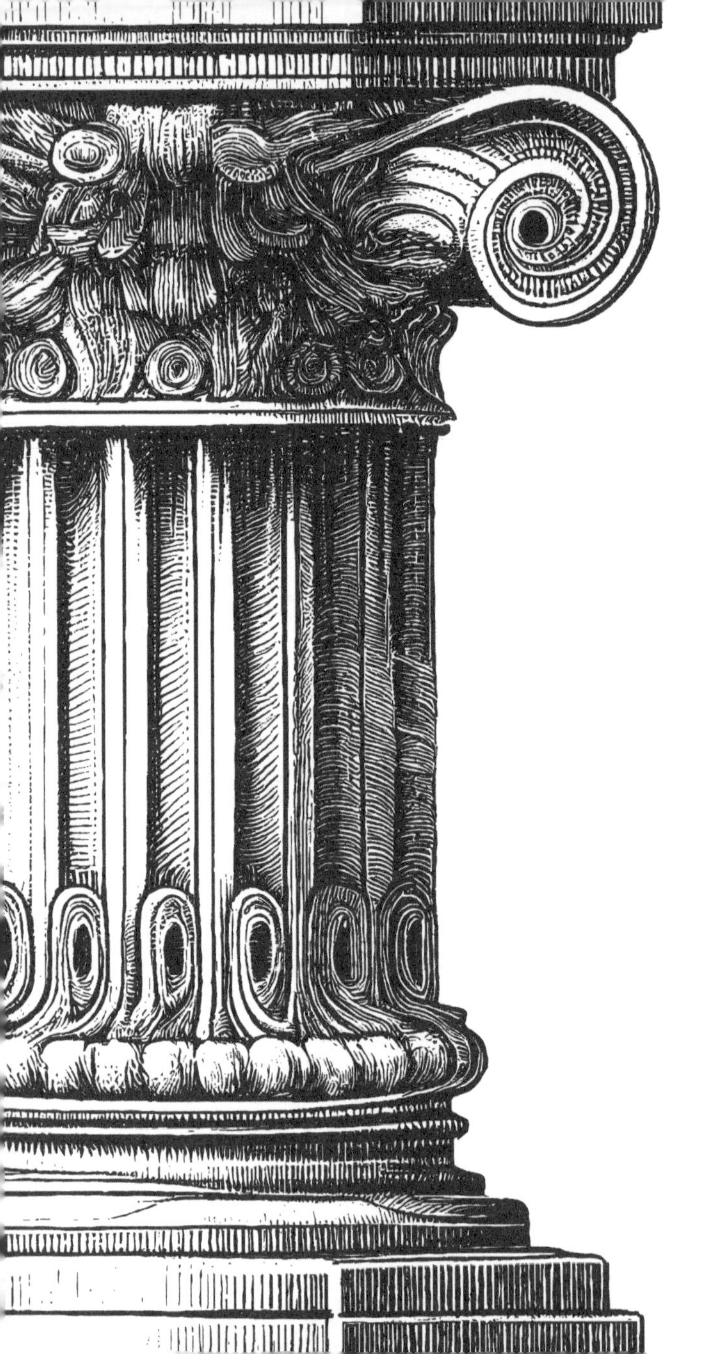

VI

MENTAL HEALTH

THE WORDS OF THE greatest Stoic philosophers offer you a timeless guide to overall better mental health. The wisdom and virtues embraced through Stoicism helps you maintain a positive and optimistic mindset while grounding you in reality and realistic expectations. These Stoic quotes provide a practical guide on how to approach life's challenges with a calm, rational, and resilient mindset.

The teachings of Stoicism encourage you to focus on what you can control, accept what you can't, and maintain a sense of inner peace regardless of external circumstances.This state of mind fosters strong mental health. Life is full of inevitable challenges and setbacks, but how you respond to them is what matters. Developing the ability to accept adversity with an open mind can improve emotional resilience.

Stoics believe negative emotions come not from the event itself but from how you perceive and react to it. Learning to reframe negative thoughts can help alleviate unwanted and sometimes unneeded emotional distress. The importance of cultivating acceptance and contentment from within, rather than relying on external circumstances to determine your happiness is the key to mental health. Daily self-reflection on your thoughts, emotions, and reactions can stimulate self-growth and overall well-being. Use these quotes as a starting point to help you on your journey to Stoicism and wellness.

STOIC STRATEGIES FOR MENTAL HEALTH

Practice Mindfulness: Stoicism emphasizes the importance of being present. Practicing mindfulness by fully engaging in the current moment without distraction allows you to manage stress and avoid overthinking.

Change Your Focus: Practice self-discipline by being in control of your behaviors and thoughts. Make a list of those things that are within your control versus those which are not. Focus only on what is within your control while letting go of what is not.

Reframe Your Thinking: Change your perspective of situations by viewing them with an optimistic lens. View challenges as potential learning opportunities. This helps turn obstacles into opportunities for growth and reduces the emotional distress accompanied by difficult experiences.

"You have power over your mind—not outside events. Realize this, and you will find strength."

—MARCUS AURELIUS

"He who indulges empty fears earns himself real fears."

—SENECA

"The happiness of your life depends upon the quality of your thoughts."

—MARCUS AURELIUS

"Man is disturbed not by things, but by the views he takes of them."

—EPICTETUS

"Very little is needed to make a happy life; it is all within yourself, in your way of thinking."

—MARCUS AURELIUS

"We should always allow some time to elapse, for time discloses the truth."

—SENECA

"In the first place, do not allow yourself to be carried away by the intensity of your impression: but say, 'Impression, wait for me a little. Let me see what you are, and what you represent. Let me test you.' Then, afterwards, do not allow it to draw you on by picturing what may come next, for if you do, it will lead you wherever it pleases. But rather, you should introduce some fair and noble impression to replace it, and banish this base and sordid one."

—EPICTETUS

"You will earn the respect of all men if you begin by earning the respect of yourself."

—MUSONIUS RUFUS

"We must have these principles ready to hand. Without them we must do nothing. We must set our mind on this object: pursue nothing that is outside us, nothing that is not our own, even as He that is mighty has ordained: pursuing what lies within our will [prohairetika], and all else [i.e., indifferent things] only so far as it is given to us. Further, we must remember who we are, and by what name we are called, and must try to direct our acts [kathêkonta] to fit each situation and its possibilities."

—EPICTETUS

"To be calm is the highest achievement of the self."

—ZEN PROVERB INSPIRED BY STOIC PRINCIPLES

"We must consider what is the time for singing, what the time for play, and in whose presence: what will be unsuited to the occasion; whether our companions are to despise us, or we to despise ourselves: when to jest, and whom to mock at: in a word, how one ought to maintain one's character in society. Wherever you swerve from any of these principles, you suffer loss at once; not loss from without, but issuing from the very act itself."

—EPICTETUS

"The human being is born with an inclination toward virtue."

—MUSONIUS RUFUS

"You must completely control your desire and shift your avoidance to what lies within your reasoned choice. You must no longer feel anger, resentment, envy, or regret."

—EPICTETUS

"If you accomplish something good with hard work, the labor passes quickly, but the good endures; if you do something shameful in pursuit of pleasure, the pleasure passes quickly, but the shame endures."

—MUSONIUS RUFUS

"The greatest remedy for anger is delay."

—SENECA

"First say to yourself what you would be; and then do what you have to do."

—EPICTETUS

"We are more often frightened than hurt, and we suffer more from imagination than from reality."

—SENECA

"I can at once become happy anywhere, for he is happy who has found himself a happy lot. In a word, happiness lies all in the functions of reason, in warrantable desires and virtuous practice."

—MARCUS AURELIUS

"I, Brutus, being the daughter of Cato, was given to you in marriage, not like a concubine, to partake only in the common intercourse of bed and board, but to bear a part in all your good and all your evil fortunes; and for your part, as regards your care for me, I find no reason to complain; but from me, what evidence of my love, what satisfaction can you receive, if I may not share with you in bearing your hidden griefs, nor to be admitted to any of your counsels that require secrecy and trust? I know very well that women seem to be of too weak a nature to be trusted with secrets; but certainly, Brutus, a virtuous birth and education, and the company of the good and honorable, are of some force to the forming our manners; and I can boast that I am the daughter of Cato, and the wife of Brutus, in which two titles though before I put less confidence, yet now I have tried myself, and find that I can bid defiance to pain."

—PORCIA CATONIS, TO HER HUSBAND AFTER A SELF-INFLICTED WOUND

"Happiness is the realization of one's wishes; but the standard is not man's ignorance but the nature of the thing."

—CHRYSIPPUS

"The happiness of your life depends upon the quality of your thoughts: therefore, guard accordingly, and take care that you entertain no notions unsuitable to virtue and reasonable nature."

—MARCUS AURELIUS

"Remember that very little is needed to make a happy life; it is all in yourself, in your way of thinking."

—MARCUS AURELIUS

"An angry man opens his mouth and shuts his eyes."

—CATO

"True happiness is to enjoy the present, without anxious dependence upon the future, not to amuse ourselves with either hopes or fears but to rest satisfied with what we have, which is sufficient, for he who is so wants nothing. The greatest blessings of mankind are within us and within our reach. A wise man is content with his lot, whatever it may be, without wishing for what he has not."

—SENECA

"Cowards die many times before their death."

—JULIUS CAESAR

"The happiness of those who want to be popular depends on others; the happiness of those who seek pleasure fluctuates with moods outside their control; but the happiness of the wise grows out of their own free acts."

—MARCUS AURELIUS

"To relax your mind…is to lose it."

—MUSONIUS RUFUS

"Be indifferent to what makes no difference."

—MARCUS AURELIUS

"Such as bathing appears to you—oil, sweat, dirt, filthy water, all things disgusting—so is every part of life and everything."

—MARCUS AURELIUS

"A man is as miserable as he thinks he is."

—SENECA

"Willingly accept the inevitable, and you will lead a life in harmony with the universe."

—MUSONIUS RUFUS

"Reflect on how many things have happened that you didn't want, and yet they turned out for the best."

—MUSONIUS RUFUS

"If you really want to escape the things that harass you, what you're needing is not to be in a different place but to be a different person."

—SENECA

"Happiness is a good flow of life."

—ZENO OF CITIUM

"Do not spoil what you have by desiring what you have not; remember that what you now have was once among the things you only hoped for."

—EPICURUS

"Above all things, respect yourself."

—PYTHAGORAS

"We can easily forgive a child who is afraid of the dark; the real tragedy of life is when men are afraid of the light."

—PLATO

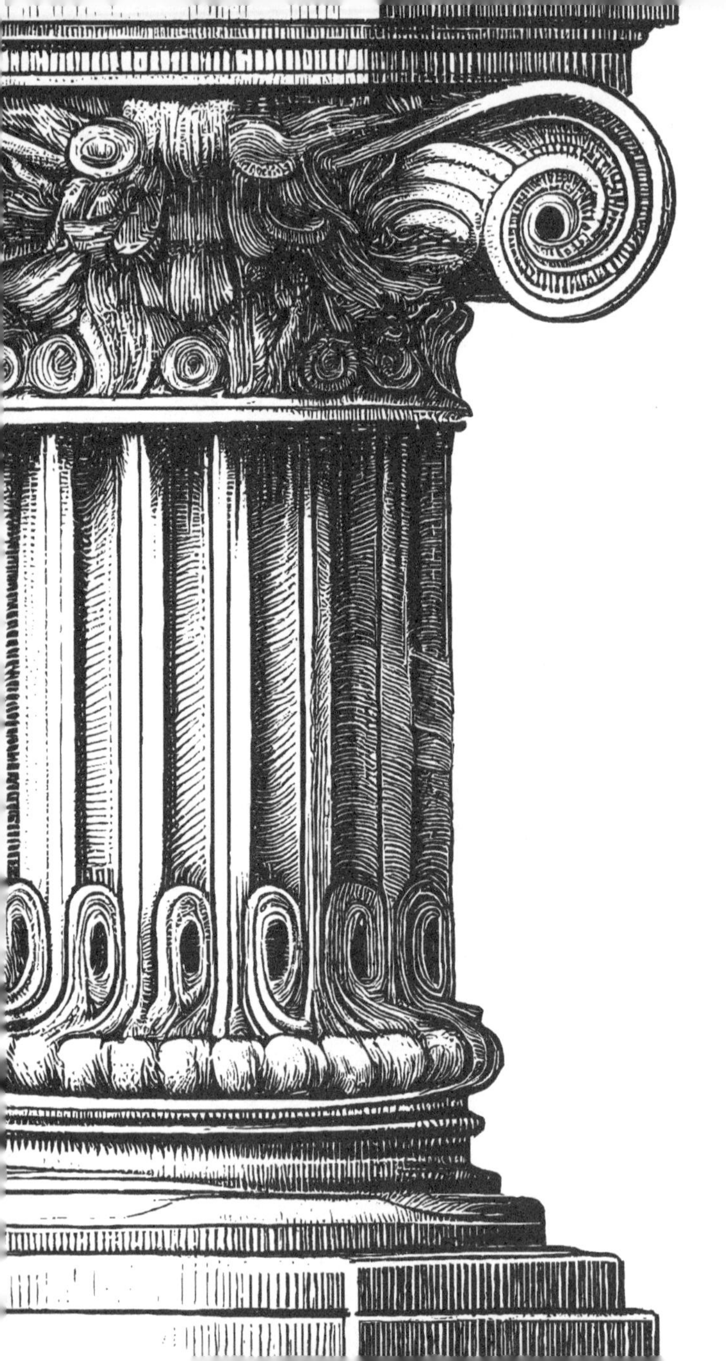

VII

BALANCE

LIVING IN BALANCE IS the ultimate goal for a Stoic. Stoicism emphasizes balance in life and living in harmony with nature, which encompasses both the natural world and human nature. By living a virtuous life, the Stoics believe that finding balance is achievable but takes practice. The use of self-reflection, rational thinking, and self-improvement can help you find balance. Seneca's writings stress the significance of "enough" and the importance of living a well-balanced life.

Stoics view balance as an ongoing practice of aligning one's behaviors and attitude with reason and acceptance. True balance in life is found in accepting what you cannot control and thoughtfully choosing your responses. Rational thinking, rather than emotionally impulsive behaviors, will allow you to achieve inner peace and balance. Make it a goal to find equilibrium within yourself and your actions, and to cope with life's challenges using a resilient mindset.

While Stoics strive to live in balance they are, however, inherently aware of the fact that life is unpredictable. Acknowledging and accepting this belief is what helps Stoics adapt and change when needed. Seeking wisdom in your actions and reacting based on thought and reason affords you the emotional balance needed to live a virtuous life. Living in balance and avoiding extremes regarding your emotions and actions allows you to maintain a rational approach to life.

STOIC STRATEGIES FOR BALANCE

Self-Reflect: Ask yourself daily if you have responded with rationality and reason. Did you have control over your reactions, or could you have reacted more thoughtfully?

Acceptance: Remind yourself that change is inevitable and a part of life. View change as an integral part of nature and accept what you cannot control.

Use Positive Thinking: Regularly reflect on the positive aspects of your life and be thankful for what you have rather than focusing on what you don't have.

"Imagine that the keeper of a huge, strong beast notices what makes it angry, what it desires, how it has to be approached and handled, the circumstances and the conditions under which it becomes particularly fierce or calm, what provokes its typical cries, and what tones of voice make it gentle or wild. Once he's spent enough time in the creature's company to acquire all this information, he calls it knowledge, forms it into a systematic branch of expertise, and starts to teach it, despite total ignorance, in fact, about which of the creature's attitudes and desires is commendable or deplorable, good, or bad, moral or immoral. His usage of all these terms simply conforms to the great beast's attitudes, and he describes things as good or bad according to its likes and dislikes, and can't justify his usage of the terms any further, but describes as right and good the things which are merely indispensable, since he hasn't realized and can't explain to anyone else how vast a gulf there is between necessity and goodness."

—PLATO, *THE REPUBLIC*

"The art of living is more like wrestling than dancing."

—MARCUS AURELIUS

"From my government Verus [I learned] good morals and the government of my temper."

—MARCUS AURELIUS

"Moderation is the key to everything."

—EPICTETUS

"The tranquility that comes when you stop caring what they say. Or think or do. Only what you do."

—MARCUS AURELIUS

"Son, remember your courage with each step."

—A SPARTAN MOTHER TO HER SON

"He has the most who is content with the least."

—DIOGENES LAËRTIUS

"We have two ears and one mouth, so we should listen more than we say."

—EPICTETUS

"Live in harmony with nature."

—ZENO OF CITIUM

"Every hour, focus your mind attentively… on the performance of the task in hand, with dignity, human sympathy, benevolence and freedom, and leave aside all other thoughts. You will achieve this, if you perform each action as if it were your last."

—MARCUS AURELIUS

"I begin to speak only when I'm certain what I'll say isn't better left unsaid."

—CATO

"Be kind, for everyone you meet is fighting a harder battle."

—PLATO

"Have I done something for the common good? Then I share in the benefits."

—MARCUS AURELIUS

"A room without books is like a body without a soul."

—CICERO

"Some things are up to us and some things are not up to us. Our opinions are up to us, and our impulses, desires, aversions—in short, whatever is our own doing. Our bodies are not up to us, nor are our possessions, our reputations, or our public offices, or, that is, whatever is not our own doing."

—EPICTETUS

"Gratitude is not only the greatest of virtues, but the parent of all others."

—CICERO

"When a dog is tied to a cart, if it wants to follow, it is pulled and follows, making its spontaneous act coincide with necessity. But if the dog does not follow, it will be compelled in any case. So it is with men to; even if they don't want to, they will be compelled to follow what is destined."

—ZENO OF CITIUM

"Dogs and philosophers do the greatest good and get the fewest rewards."

—DIOGENES LAËRTIUS

"He who has equipped himself for the whole of life does not need to be advised concerning each separate thing, because he is now trained to meet his problem as a whole; for he knows not merely how he should live with his wife or his son, but how he should live aright."

—ARISTOTLE

"It is not the man who has too little, but the man who craves more, that is poor."

—SENECA

"First learn the meaning of what you say, and then speak."

—EPICTETUS

"No plague has cost the human race more dear: you will see slaughterings and poisonings, accusations and counter-accusations, sacking of cities, ruin of whole peoples, the persons of princes sold into slavery by auction, torches applied to roofs, and fires not merely confined within city-walls but making whole tracts of country glow with hostile flame."

—SENECA

"If I followed the multitude, I should not have studied philosophy."

—CHRYSIPPUS

"How much better to heal than seek revenge from injury. Vengeance wastes a lot of time and exposes you to many more injuries than the first that sparked it. Anger always outlasts hurt. Best to take the opposite course."

—SENECA

"Whoever then understands what is good, can also know how to love; but he who cannot distinguish good from bad, and things which are neither good nor bad from both, can he possess the power of loving? To love, then, is only in the power of the wise."

—SENECA

"A single day among the learned lasts longer than the longest life of the ignorant."

—POSIDONIUS

"To be ignorant of what occurred before you were born is to remain always a child."

—CICERO

"As a matter of self-perseveration, a man needs good friends or ardent enemies, for the former instruct him and the latter take him to task."

—DIOGENES LAËRTIUS

"Six mistakes mankind keeps making century after century:

Believing that personal gain is made by crushing others;

Worrying about things that cannot be changed or corrected;

Insisting that a thing is impossible because we cannot accomplish it;

Refusing to set aside trivial preferences;

Neglecting development and refinement of the mind;

Attempting to compel others to believe and live as we do."

—CICERO

"Love is born into every human being; it calls back the halves of our original nature together; it tries to make one out of two and heal the wound of human nature."

—PLATO

Final Thoughts

In the end, Stoicism reminds us that true strength lies not in what we control, but in how we meet what we cannot. When the mind is calm, the body follows; when the body is cared for, the mind finds clarity. The Stoics taught that a sound mind and a healthy body are not separate pursuits, but parts of the same whole. By tending to both with wisdom, discipline, and gratitude, we live not just longer, but better. To live well is to align the mind and body with nature's rhythm, breathing deeply, thinking clearly, and acting justly until well-being becomes our way of life.

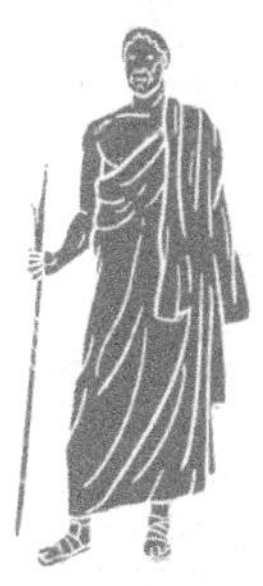

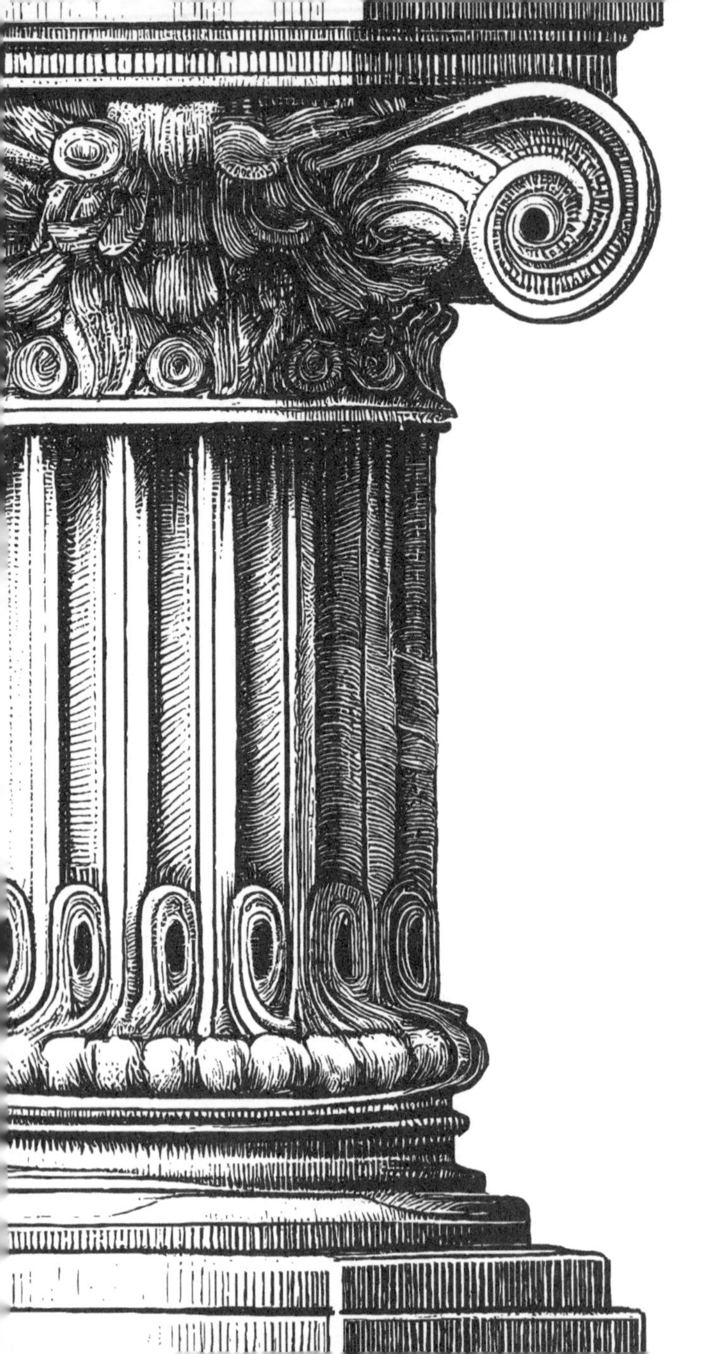

About the Authors

Nick Benas grew up in Guilford, Connecticut. A former United States Marine Sergeant and Iraq Combat Veteran, Nick is a 2nd Dan Black Belt in Tae Kwon-Do and a Green Belt Instructor in the Marine Corps Martial Arts Program. He holds an undergraduate degree in Sociology and an MS in Public Policy from Southern Connecticut State University. He has been featured for his business success and entrepreneurship by more than 50 major media outlets, including Entrepreneur Magazine, Men's Health, ABC, FOX, ESPN, and CNBC. His passion lies in serving veterans and writing.

Kortney Yasenka, LCMHC, is a licensed clinical mental health counselor who provides individual, family, and group therapy, as well as life coaching services. Kortney is certified in trauma-focused cognitive behavioral therapy and incorporates physical activity and eco-therapy into counseling and coaching sessions. She has a Masters in Counseling Psychology with a concentration in Health Psychology from

Northeastern University. With over 20 years of experience, Kortney has worked in community mental health, school systems, and private practice. In her free time, she enjoys running, spending time with family, and vacationing on the beautiful island of St. John. Find more of Kortney at kortneyyasenka.com and yasenkacounseling.com.

Also by Nick Benas

The Marcus Aurelius Book of Quotes
The Stoicism Book of Quotes
The Warrior's Book of Virtues
The Resilient Warrior
Warrior Wisdom
Tactical Mobility
Mental Health Emergencies

Also by Kortney Yasenka

The Marcus Aurelius Book of Quotes
The Stoicism Book of Quotes
Swedish Lagom

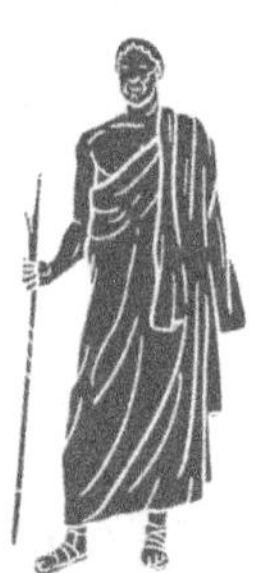